A NUMB CONVERSATION
& THE PLACE BETWEEN TWO SIDES

WRITTEN BY
M. HUNTER & AMINA HUNTER

Michael Terence
Publishing

First published in paperback by
Michael Terence Publishing in 2020
www.mtp.agency

ISBN 9781800940208

Cover image
by M. Hunter

Interior image
Copyright © M. Hunter

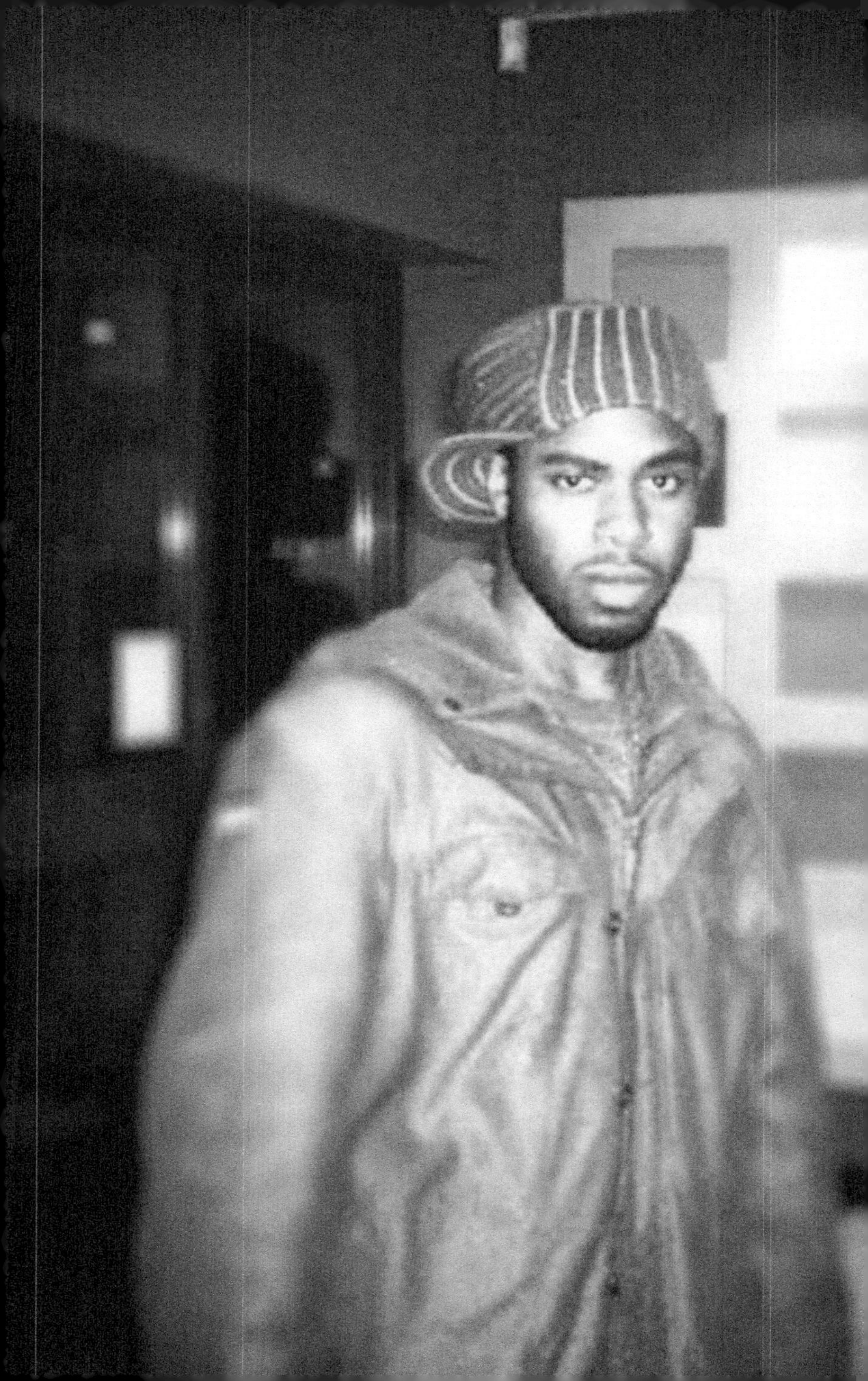

Contents

Prologue

My name is Mohammad Hunter; Moe for short, but my family calls me 'Muki'. This is my story.

It was summer 2003. I was perched on the windowsill in the backroom of my house. Linkin Park's Meteora album was playing in the background. I had a Nintendo GameCube controller in my hand and I was playing Wave Race: Blue Storm, trying to beat Abdullah's, my younger brother, high score.

I could remember thinking how perfect that moment was, not even just that moment, but my whole life. I had a great job, amazing friends and a loving family - all the things I could've asked for. Life was literally in my hands – until it suddenly slipped through my grasp and left me…

My house was a pit stop where fun was found, had and remembered. Abdullah and I, along with some friends, would have late-night gaming sessions on our Nintendo GameCubes, always left feeling like we could do anything; be anyone.

My life was soaring, fun-filled and full of endless opportunities…

…until illness soon came and replaced opportunity with obstacles.

Let me take you to the place where my battle began, and memory ended.

Summer merged into Autumn as I sat in my home studio looking through a movie magazine with a feature on the Lord of the Rings - Return of the King. I'd been eagerly anticipating it!

Autumn merged into winter and brought December 2003 with it. I celebrated my 20th Birthday and got to watch the entire Lord of the Rings trilogy that day. It was one of the greatest years of my life; the life that blessed me with happiness and contentment.

Though, little did I know, that my contentment would soon be gone. Can you really have a life where there is happiness without sadness, light without dark, life without death? This journey can change direction in a heartbeat. *It* doesn't care if you're happy or not.

It'll still form grey clouds above you on the sunniest of days. And it was those clouds that engulfed me and dumped rain showers down with fury. And so, the year came to an end; as did my memory.

Before the numbness

It was the year 2019, I was sat with my Mom telling her my decision to write about my personal journey. I wanted to write everything down, as my memory is not as reliable as it once was. My illness went outside of just being physical and became an emotional torment for my family.

I heavily relied on my Mother's memory to fill in the blanks. Her perspective helped complete the complexity of emotions, feelings and events that took place - events that are so numb in conversation - the one that took place between her and me, was one that will stay etched in my memory for the rest of my life.

This was a time where I was lost but she never stopped searching, hoping, praying for me to return. Our conversation proved to be deeply emotional, and although both in the same place at the same time, we were on two completely different paths that had become disconnected through no choice of our own.

For the last time in my life, I was back in a coma, while we revisited and spoke of my past.

Let's start with my Mother's side of the story…

A Mother's pain is her son's numbness

August 2004 was a life-changing month. I didn't know at that time that this would become a significant date, neither did I know that my son would be the reason for it.

After two weeks in Benidorm, Spain, I returned home to Birmingham to find Moe with a cough. I thought it strange as he was rarely sick. It was a persistent cough – a cough that turned (maybe) only a Mother's head? I didn't give it all my attention, but it was enough of a cough to keep grabbing my attention.

On the last Thursday in August (despite the cough), Moe and his younger siblings went to Perry Park summer fair and were gone the entire day.

They all arrived back just a little before sunset, which was a typical routine for their return home. They were all in my bedroom filling me in on the day at the fair, but I noticed something was off. Albeit, a normal recount of the day's events, Moe was far from normal in his demeanour. At first, I thought it was due to the exhilaration of the day's events, and that he was finding it hard to get his words out. I asked him what was wrong, but there was an emptiness to the words that were tumbling out of his mouth. I could not make sense of his words, or the situation that was unfolding.

Humour can overtake emotions in times of shock. This is what must have happened, as we awkwardly laughed at his responses. Things took a dramatic and serious tone when I realized he was genuinely struggling to form a proper sentence, or even get his words out. To add to my growing concern, his eyes began flickering and the atmosphere became heavy and not-one-bit humorous. He couldn't focus on anything and began to fit.

On his knees, leaning against my bed, I tried to be a calming influence, telling him to breathe properly and speak slowly. My heart sank deep into that reserved pit that only a Mother can explain. Despite my fear, I kept my composure and stayed calm; the only gift I could give him.

Again, he tried telling me what was happening to him, but his speech was slurred, the more he tried, the more incomprehensible it became. The digestion of seeing such a familiar face, lost in such an unfamiliar body had a bitter taste. The capable, twenty-year-old son who was talking yesterday, simply couldn't be heard today - My son.

My heart was heavy. A paralyzing fear had surfaced - the fear (along with impatience) was suffocating, slowly taking control. How could I make sense of something that made no sense at all? I became annoyed with Moe, telling him to 'speak properly!'. In retrospect, I can honestly say, I was just desperate to hear him speak normally. My heart was breaking. I didn't know a Mum could hold her breath for so long. There is no doubt about it, I wanted to stay in denial, this was a much safer place. What was the alternative?

Moe being without voice, lead me to reach for a pen and paper for him to explain what was happening. I ordered him to write his unspoken words, but that didn't help or work. He started writing in a straight line but that line wavered as if he was making a graph of some kind. His attempts to write were mere scribbles, it was at this point that I realized I'd still been holding my breath. I could feel a hard lump in my throat; fear? Gut instinct? In hindsight, I'd like to think it was the latter.

I leaned in close to calm him. He wasn't the best writer to begin with, but his struggle to write the simplest line was as real as his effort in trying. Everything he wrote was as indecipherable as the attempts of a two-year-old.

"What's wrong with you, Muks? Write properly! Write what you're trying to say!" I remember saying.

He looked across at me with his big puppy dog eyes that held a solemn sadness - new and foreign to my sight. He agreed to do his best with sincerity and endeavoured to put the pen to a paper once more. His effort simply wasn't enough, and it was clear that this was out of his control. All the willingness in the world wouldn't change the outcome. If he wasn't in control; I certainly wasn't in control. Lost in my worry; all sorts of irrational thoughts were flooding in. I couldn't focus, couldn't comprehend what was happening to my son. One minute he was fine, and the next, he was lost to an overpowering force that couldn't be seen. I could hardly breathe for the fear that had enveloped me.

All this time, his younger siblings kept encouraging him to speak and write. I have no idea if they had grasped just how serious things were becoming. Not only was his speech slurred, but he was also running a fever. Everything was moving fast, yet the world was standing still. I was thinking of ways to bring down his temperature, so I ran a lukewarm bath, added rosemary and thyme, and helped him in.

I left him to soak in the water for some time - time for me to think rationally. Maintaining my composure was paramount, I didn't want the younger children to see the worry that was trying to engulf me. My years have taught me patience in the face of life's unpredictable adversities, and as I have always taken care of my children through sickness and health, I didn't think to call the doctor at that time. This was likely both denial and desperation from a Mother to her child. A last attempt at gaining back some control.

I settled him down, for what was a very restless night. Mothers are probably the only people that have a skill of peripheral vision. We can sleep with eyes open and ears that are alerted to the slightest of noise from her child.

He was extremely agitated throughout the night and my eyes were on him with every movement he made. His temperature was soaring. We got through the night with very little sleep and contrary to my previous hope for being the one to Mother him back to health, I admitted defeat and took him to the doctor.

After a brief examination, the doctor diagnosed him with a throat infection and prescribed a course of antibiotics. I saw something deep within Moe's eyes that spoke louder than any word he had spoken whilst unwell. The decision to take him home did not sit comfortably with me, but I had no rational reason to object. I am not a massive believer in conventional medicines, and I believe in them even less, when they are distributed to clear a doctor's busy schedule.

I gave the antibiotics, mainly because there was nothing else to give. I became even more concerned when he showed no improvement by the end of the day. He was deteriorating regardless of tablets, and by the Saturday he was slipping in and out of consciousness. His facial expressions were creating movements I had never seen before. The loudness in his eyes kept peering out at me. The inner child reaching out for his Mum - I rang 999.

The ambulance came after an eternal (probably minutes) wait and took him to the hospital. Upon reaching Dudley road A&E, we received a non-urgent colour-coded card. The hospital staff were inundated with what appeared to be the 'usual crowd' expected on a weekend. All this time, unbeknown to me, or the triage nurse (who had made the decision to downgrade the urgency to him being seen) the shadow of death was calling my son. The truly unwell patients can be the quietest.

It was over an hour before a doctor finally entered the cubicle. After explaining what had been happening to Moe, starting with his onset of symptoms and the most recent GP diagnosis, the doctor proceeded to examine him. First, the stethoscope, then some blood for testing, an ear check, then he dismissed himself. I can't even remember him introducing himself. Funny how minor details can stay etched in your memory, like the pattern on the hospital screen, or the name of the screaming child in the next cubicle, but not the name of an important doctor that misdiagnosed your child.

After more hours of waiting, that doctor returned with the questionable diagnosis of an ear infection. I remember feeling hopeless and almost invisible. We left the hospital with a new diagnosis and arrived home at 3am on Sunday.

I walked into the house with a willingness to try the antibiotics, along with the most effective form of medicine I have ever had to hand - prayer. I knew, deep in my soul, that there was something seriously wrong with my son, and that only God would highlight it. We might not be certified physicians, but Mothers are the best at knowing when things are not right with their children. It's a physical and spiritual connection that God created. I knew in my heart that this was only the beginning of something far, far worse.

With no improvement by the Monday, I decided to take him back to the hospital. By this point, Moe was delirious and still running a fever. The words that were being mumbled days before, were now silent. My worry was swirling in a hollow, empty space in the pit of my stomach, where thoughts get lost, feelings are numb, and a physical pain fills the void where fulfilment once lay. This is something that every parent with a sick child knows and understands all too well.

We eventually got called to triage and were told to wait in the reception area. After five long hours of despair, seeing other people in need of doctors being treated, and sent home, whilst we still sat patiently waiting to be seen, my patience left my side and I suggested for us to go home.

Time was passing us by, along with everyone else being seen, but us. Another taxi drive later, we were back home. I helped Moe to bed, and I prayed – prayed hard. We had another very restless night.

Just before noon on the Tuesday, sunbeams shone over him, and he got out of bed. A promising sound, until he stumbled across the floor, and with that followed a sickening thud. I leapt out of bed to find my son collapsed on the floor, no sunbeams in sight.

I couldn't make any sense out of what he was trying to say. I rushed to the phone and dialled 999 for the second time that week. I explained what had happened to the operator and before I ended the call, the paramedics were knocking at my door. Leaving him in the hands of my faith, I rushed downstairs and let the ambulance men in. I led them upstairs to Moe on the floor. They asked a few questions, examined him thoroughly and that instigated him being carted off in the ambulance back to where he should have been.

Moe was semi-conscious and unable to make himself clear. When we got to the hospital, I signed him in at reception while they wheeled him straight through to the back of the hospital. After finishing at reception, I joined him where we were left in an open area exposed to the sick and injured. We were there for quite some time with Moe sat in the wheelchair as I stood behind him. We watched doctors and nurses on the computer, otherwise occupied. We were no more visible than the dust in the air. They seemed busy without a sense of urgency about them. 'Unwell' did not seem urgent enough for him to be noticed.

All was not lost. God came through. I believe he sent a beautiful doctor dressed in pale blue who noticed him - like really noticed him. She didn't hesitate in helping and she was the beginning of the end.

"This young man doesn't look well at all. Take him into the cubicle. Let me have a look at him!" were her words.

Someone (I don't recall who) wheeled him into the first cubicle and helped Moe onto the bed. By then he was not my familiar son. He kept talking nonsense, telling people that he loved them, amongst other bizarre and out of character things.

When the Heaven-sent doctor returned, she began examining him and she questioned his mental state. She did, however, see something in the back of his eyes that raised enough concern to call for a second opinion.

"Is he always like this?" The other newly arrived female doctor asked.

"I don't know this person. That is not my son!" I told them. "How long has he been like this?" She asked.

"Since Thursday." And I explained exactly what had transpired since they returned from the fair, right up to this point, this very scary, surreal point. I watched them closely as they tried to reach a conclusion as to what they were; and weren't seeing. A stroke was mentioned at one stage, but he could move all his limbs. Then came that crucial moment when they tried to get him to lift and bend his leg, and he gave out a harrowing scream.

That scream will haunt me forever. What was once just a fear of possibilities, were now actual happening took my fear to a whole new level.

Things moved up a gear and the sea of doctors became like waves in a storm. This snapshot is where I saw doctors come to life and work in their prime. Fear also moved them; not like a Mother's fear, because that is paralyzing – fear moves their thoughts, their actions and they come to life; ironically, as my son was losing his. Time really does stand still in the wake of disaster. Bloodwork wasn't highlighting what was going on with Moe, which was sending the doctors back into their experiences, trying to trace similar symptoms that could lead to a diagnosis.

I prayed.

The woman who birthed a son on the 13th of December 1983, at the Sorento maternity hospital in Moseley, prayed then, and I prayed 20 years later for the same thing. I wanted my baby to survive.

Moe was kept in on the critical care unit. That word 'critical' will not resonate on the severity of the situation. It still sends shock waves through me when I say the word out loud. My child was in 'critical' condition, with what appeared to be an unknown condition, with an unknown treatment and an unknown outcome.

"We're going to get to the bottom of what is wrong with your son. We will do more tests and a lumbar punch, where we take some of the fluid from the spine to test it." The doctor was speaking, but his words weren't reaching me. I could take the words in, but not the meaning.

I have no idea what time scales were at that time. Minutes may have been hours, and hours may have been minutes. I am certain that time stood still too. I stayed with Moe all night. A decision that no Mother is comfortable with when choosing between her children, forcing her to be with the one in most need.

Diagnosing the numbness

How are the quietest words the loudest? TB.

Those were the quiet whispers I heard on my return – Tuberculosis.

My son was situated in the corner of the ward, completely out of place. This was not where he belonged. Seeing something as familiar as your heartbeat, in an unfamiliar surrounding is too surreal. I couldn't bear to see him become unfamiliar too.

Wednesday brought a new face. Not one I remember fondly. It amazed me how one doctor could seem like they were born to do a job, yet other doctors were merely doing a job because they'd been born; no in-between, black and white. Even before she had crossed the threshold into the room, she had made a judgement about my son, just like I had made a judgement about her.

The young woman was empty on small talk. She was in no mood for *any* talk! She was there to do one job – lumbar puncture. I was lost for words. 'You will have to be still,' she cautioned Moe.

"Come on, Muks," I said, grabbing hold of him, folding his body into a fetal position, and keeping him there until she was successful at extracting the fluid from his spine. Seemed a fitting and appropriate position for him to be in, considering her manner.

"How long before we know anything?" I asked. Her response was as cold as her bedside manner. I prayed.

Hours passed in silent thoughts and worry.

The results came in with a person that was the complete opposite to the last. There was sympathy in her eye. A disconnected look of sorrow compared to her cold exterior earlier. She wasn't just here to 'do a job', she was here to deliver bad news – and bad news it certainly was.

The next paragraph was not heard in this way at the time. It was muffled and noisy, but not due to loud words. I think it was my heartbeat over words, fear, panic and disbelief.

"Poor man, he is very, very ill. He has meningitis of the brain. We're going to start him on antibiotics straight away." I prayed.

They wheeled him into a ward further down the hallway where it was warm. The air felt different.

I met the neurological consultant, and he was the most gentle and kindest man I met throughout the entire experience. The doctor explained the next steps in a matter of fact way. Exactly how a Mother can make sense of words at a time of utter loss. I asked some questions, but do not remember the answers. I just remember him giving me his honest and professional medical opinion.

"There is a fifty per cent chance that the antibiotic will work, and at this stage in treatment, we cannot say what his prognosis will be, neither can we predict damage already caused…" he stopped when he saw fear rise up in me. Respectfully, he retracted from the rest of his sentence and allowed me time to sieve through facts, emotion, fear, panic, hope and prayer.

I returned home to prepare his siblings. "Muks is very ill. He has meningitis of the brain and the doctors say he has a fifty per cent chance of surviving." This news was quite possibly the most bizarre news. Hope and no hope all in one sentence.

I went on to say - "You see, he doesn't belong to us; he belongs to God. I am just a vessel by which God brought him into this world and if God sees fit to take him, we say 'Alhamdulillah', but we hope and pray that he will leave him with us for a little while longer."

We fell into each other's arms and cried.

When I returned to the hospital, although my children's pain and confusion still with me, my entire being was detached, closed to everything else, but Moe. Prayer was my only deliverance, in it I found comfort, hope and faith.

Fifty / fifty

I didn't feel conscious, I was desperately clinging onto my faith. This storm just didn't feel real. Ironically, it was very real because on my return home, red river burst her banks and she raged for a full month.

Treatment started on Thursday, as did his coma.

I had the task of informing family members of his situation, that took courage and strength; breathing life into the reality of the status he was in. Kind words and support simply did not reach my despair.

I refer to this time as a 'triangle'. The points represented me, Moe and God all inside the triangle, reaching for one another; everything and everyone else was on the outside.

Looking back, there was a dream I had whilst pregnant that resurfaced and projected emotions, stirring my current worries.

A few weeks before going into labour, I dreamt of giving birth to a beautiful boy, with loose tousled hair and attached to his curls were eggshells.

Now, here I am 20 years later, staring at my beautiful boy – my baby – walking on eggshells, being mindful of his fragile state and the fifty per cent chance of him surviving, with the unthinkable other fifty per cent alternative - too delicate to consider. Do I love him harder, or retract to prepare for letting him go?

This is a Mother's numbness to love.

By Saturday, Moe was still in a coma. He had been moved to ward D46, which wasn't exactly a hotel room. There were no obvious signs of the antibiotics working. I stayed by his bedside; a quiet and lonely place. Of course, people came and went, returning to their normal lives. When I returned home, it was to take care of duties and jobs. Rest would have been ideal, but my thoughts and worries travelled by my side, whether I was at the hospital or at home. The evening I did settle down for some sleep was interrupted with a call.

"Hello, is this Mrs Hunter?" the female voice asked.
"Yes," I said.

"I am calling from the hospital. Moe is okay, but we need you to come in and look after him, we have no-one watching over him."

I don't remember whether she mentioned her name, all I can recall was my heart skipping a beat and making a rhythm of its own. I took a deep breath and told them I would be with them as soon as I could.

Over time I realized that he really was a hindrance to the staff. The ward was in no fit state for anyone other than the already passed, making the experience all the more depressing and distressing. Sunday morning, the doctors visited and with an obvious sign of him not doing well, he requested an MRI. The result was another blow to the heart. His brain was swelling, and the hospital couldn't accommodate his condition. He was to be transferred to the QE.

"The QE is the only place adequate and equipped to deal with his neurological condition. We will arrange for him to go there immediately. Unfortunately, this is a matter of life and death!" The doctor said.

I broke down and cried inconsolably. The ground I was relying on to keep me on my feet had suddenly been pulled from under me.

When he arrived at the QE, I was given a yellow consent form. This was to give consent to life-saving brain surgery. It was explained how the operation would take three hours and they needed to put a shunt in his head. I had no idea what this was or meant, my mind was still stuck on the fallen words of 'life-saving'. I trusted in God (and the doctor) and held onto that faith with hope and prayer. For the first time since Thursday, I felt there was a shift in the bleakness. I instinctively knew he would survive.

His life would be saved. I believed God had heard my prayers.

I sat in that waiting room with some other people. A Canadian Christian lady was there for her longstanding friend. I later learned that she had travelled all the way from Canada to see her dearest friend, only to end up at the hospital after she suffered a stroke during her visit. There was also the Mom and Dad who were sitting apart and didn't pass any words to each other. The blame of their sons attempted suicide was lay at the Mum's doorstep, placed there by the Dad. I felt her pain, as not only was her son on life support, but she was suffering the blame too. When I saw their son, he was on every machine imaginable. It was hard to imagine him ever recovering. The Mum had a hollowness to her eyes, possibly where she was tirelessly searching for all the 'what ifs and whys'.

"Do you believe in God?" I remember asking her. "Well, I used to, but I don't know now," she answered.

"Don't lose faith in hope. Your son will be fine. Just

trust in the Almighty God!" I told her. The Christian lady from Canada gave a nod of approval and agreement in my statement.

Then, there was the Mother whose baby was in intensive care. She was extremely distraught.

So, there we all were - three female strangers sitting in the waiting room, waiting for the only news we wanted to hear about our children. We didn't know each other, yet we consoled and comforted each other as if we were deeply connected at that time. This is humanity at its best.

Three hours stretched into four, and many times I was pacing the hallway, interrupting every nurse that passed, to ask if my son was out of theatre.

The answer was always the same and so it went on.

Four hours and fifteen minutes later, a face appeared in the doorway of the waiting room to announce the long-awaited news. The operation was a success! I could go and see him – I could see my son-alive.

The celebration of life

Almost four weeks passed from that Thursday in August, comatose all that time. The day of Moe opening his eyes was a celebration of life, just like 20 years ago. My baby opened his eyes, and I took a breath that inhaled the oxygen I had been desperate to have for weeks and exhaled the fear and worry that had weighed down my lungs for so long. I looked into his eyes, and the darkness that once consumed those beautiful eyes was gone.

A few days later they transferred him back to the Dudley road hospital, but this time, he was in a much nicer setting. I don't know whether the setting was nicer due to the setting itself, or whether it was because of Moe being in a better situation himself. He was gaunt and his skin too big for his frame, but he was alive. With a long road to recovery ahead of him, he began his journey with me by his side. Just like how he started off in life when he was born.

Moe sails his way through life's storms, always waiting for the sunshine to break. Thanks to Iks, Rim, and Ham who contributed all of their earnings to the cause.

Have you ever been stuck in between a dream, and

dreaming a dream? The place where a dream spills into the conscious mind upon waking and your mind can't decipher between what's real and what's a dream?

I could see silhouettes of people and hear a surround sound of muffled noise that strained my hearing. The lights were blinding. Catching my breath felt like an ever-escaping supply of oxygen. My vision tunnelled, the edges of my sight blurred and there seemed to be an ever-increasing darkness pulling in from the corners of my sight.

My heart was beating through my skull, pounding away reminding me I was alive. My skull felt like it was expanding and my skin stretching. There I was – awake, but dreaming maybe? As the minutes passed, I became silent. My voice trapped inside my body, and my disorientation of what was going on became more intense.

I remember being driven to say something about 'the Africans'. It made no sense and yet I had an overwhelming urge to blurt it out.

"Ask ESP about the Africans," I yelled.

Darkness was now close to blanketing my vision completely. Fear had fully wrapped its forcefulness around me, and as the darkness proceeded, my vision faded, and I entered into the other side of the world.

The lifeless garden

What some would refer to as 'my time in a coma', I refer to as 'chapters of my journey between two sides'.

I found myself standing in a garden of sundried, colourless grass. A garden lacking beauty, growth or life. This garden had no shoots of grass or budding daises. Every step created a sound of uncomfortableness. My senses were so heightened in this place. The only way I can describe it would be like wearing noise-cancelling headphones; where the echo of your own sounds was so exaggerated that they overpowered any outside noise. I could see the garden was enclosed by a six-foot fence, and as I looked further down the garden, I saw a shallow hole that had been dug. It looked as though it was filled with water but was dried up by the sun; much like the rest of the garden. I saw some familiar features that you would expect to see in a garden, but this was far from any garden that I'd ever been to. This garden was different.

I heard a tapping against the hard-dried ground, from what sounded like a dog. It was approaching me with clouds of dirt surrounding its body. I remember being unsure of the dog's symbolism. he dog walked past me, engaged my eyes and motioned me to follow it. It leads me down the garden to a Russian doll figure, dressed in black robes. Fear struck through my entire core. The figure loomed over me, making rumbling vibration sounds as it starts to approach me. The dog barked at the figure, almost like he was guarding me. Suddenly, the figure vanished back into the place he emerged from and soon after that so did the dog.

I began to feel a weird sensation, coupled with nausea. I found myself being pulled in an upward motion. Looking down, I could see my feet take off from the lifeless ground. As the garden grew smaller, my fear grew bigger as I was taken into a void of utter darkness.

In the bright blue

On the next blink, I found myself sitting on a marble surface, a huge marble stone afloat in the sky. I was submerged in blue skies, no sun in sight. The brightness appeared to be coming from an unexplainable source. It was just there; like me. This place was pure warmth. Warmth that filtered through to my soul and I felt at peace.

I heard Abdullah's voice. Another peaceful and warm sensation crept over me as I looked up and saw him beside me.

"Hey, Muk," he shouted, jumping high up into the air. He pressed his bare feet onto the marble and pushed himself off, ascending high up into the sky-blue sky. I felt a sense of happiness illuminating from inside me.

I can remember watching in awe, wondering how he was able to fly.

As he continued, I looked to the other end of this huge piece of marble and watched huge pillars erupt, rising up into the sky until I couldn't see the tops anymore. I stood up and found myself walking up a steep slope. When I reached the top, my

Mother sat on the top of a concaved wall. She smiled at me; a welcoming smile, albeit slightly dazed. Feeling content and full of my Mother's love, I fell to the abyss of the dark void once more.

The old canal

I stood on a pathway of an old, extremely eerie Victorian canal at night. An unexplainable fog plagued the air, yet my vision wasn't impaired. My physical state was stiff like I was paralyzed. I saw the canal water start to ripple as an old riverboat emerged through the fog. Next thing I know, I was on the boat and, out of nowhere, a mysterious figure appeared on the boat in front of me.

"Do not gaze upon those on the bridge," he said. I looked over my right shoulder and saw several silhouettes with bright beams of light bursting from their eyes. They were on an old, stone bridge over the far side of the canal. The figure spoke again.

"DO NOT GAZE UPON THOSE ON THE BRIDGE!"

Obliging, I turned away with haste. The boat rocked to a stop when it reached its destination. The figure mumbled something that I couldn't quite make out. To this day, I still don't know what he said. I wish I knew. It haunts me still to this day not knowing. The sun rose and my vision slipped back down through the tunnel back into darkness, leaving the macabre canal behind.

The factory

This factory looks as if it were still under construction. The atmosphere was dense with a lot of dust in the air. As I stood on an untrustworthy scaffolding, I began to scout the area. To my surprise, I saw the same black dog I encountered in the garden. It stood in a corridor with its black eyes on me. As I approached him, he began to lead me down the dark corridor.

We reached a flight of stairs and I followed the dog down them. As the last step came into sight, the dog vanished. The same figure from the lifeless garden appeared as the dog disappeared. The whole factory closed in on me like I was falling into fabric, sinking into something soft and bottomless. I sank deeper and deeper – back into the darkness that I had met too many times before…

Between two sides

Try to imagine a wall made out of earth. In the wall of earth is a hole. In that hole is fresh green grass with dew droplets from a misty summer night. A hole full of hope, life and growth, was created by this wall of earth. I called this the 'place between the two sides' because that is precisely what it was. The one side of the wall was where life started, and on the other side was where life began to grow.

From in the hole, I saw a mist-covered glass window of some sort, and to my left, the opening to this beautiful view of fields, trees, birds and colour, so enticing to the eye. A window of what beauty - what life - can offer.

I could only assume that I had died, and this was the afterlife.

I felt someone clutching at my shoulder. At the end of my shoulder, my Mother stood looking tired, sad and desperate.

"Please don't leave us, Moe, stay with us," she pleaded.

Abdullah's hand reached into the hole.

"Stay on the side of the wall, Muks," he whispered.

The temptation to want to touch the dew droplets on the grass that lay on the other side of the wall was very real. That's when I heard my Mother's cries echo around me they pulled me away from temptation.

I was on my back, surrounded by white and emptiness. I felt something foreign inside the right of my torso, just below the ribcage, I could feel something moving around inside me. I heard vibrations of voices in the distance, nothing that I could translate though. I heard loud noises and these sounds were exaggerated tenfold. I could feel so much pain and was screaming a silent plea to make it stop. A powerless moment where your voice is unheard is the most terrifying experience.

Final plain

That terrifying experience took me to a desert plain, with red cliffs all around me. As I lay down on the red rock, I felt like I was tied to it. I could feel an invisible force holding me down while I looked into the sky.

"MOHAMMAD, MOHAMMAD. It is not your time yet," my Mother's voice echoed in the sky.

I looked up and was surrounded by several figures: three faceless figures to my right, three to my left and one stood in front. They wore white robes with white, shiny pearls down the seams of the robe and had an unfamiliar symbol carved on the side of their heads.

"Mohammad it is not your time, but… we will see you again, SOON," they said in unison.

As the sun rose, the seven figures vanished. The sun rose up into the sky at an unnatural speed. Its rays beamed unbearably bright; so bright that it blinded my vision as I rose up with it back to the earth's wall.

Returning to normal

I woke up in bed at the Queen Elizabeth hospital in Birmingham, England, surrounded by my family and friends. My Mother came over. I cannot recall the first thing she or I said, but as my vision focused with my hearing, I start to hear her explain everything: that I had contracted tuberculosis and bacterial meningitis, that I had been in a coma for over a month, and that my life was saved after a VP shunt was inserted inside my brain to drain off excess fluid.

She explained the operation and how they made an incision on the right of my torso beneath the rib cage which coincided with my experience where I was in pain and had no voice. I felt unplugged from the real world, shaken.

A few days passed and I was transferred to the Birmingham city hospital. On ward D43, I was told I needed a lot of rest and rehabilitation. I was somewhat aggressive to the nurse in charge of my care. I really couldn't understand why I was feeling so out of character. I'd grown anxious, irritable, agitated and I couldn't get a good night sleep. I played Super Mario Advance on the Game Boy that my Mom had got for me, using it as a distraction, for I found myself fearful of seeing the figures that had visited me while I was gone… I still wasn't convinced that I was truly alive.

One night I thought I fell asleep but when I tried to sit up, I couldn't move. I tried to shout for a nurse, but no sound came out. I felt myself slowly rising, as if I had levitated off the bed, and was slowly descending back on to it. As I hit the bed abruptly, I inhaled a deep breath that let out a bizarre noise.

Over the next few days, when the doctor visited me, I stressed how much I wanted to go home. I felt and sounded good, so the doctor asked to see my physical abilities. I wasn't as stable as I thought I was and he denied my discharge - time seemed to drag on for what felt like an eternity.

After a week or so, I was discharged but my ordeal was not over. I had to remain an outpatient for the next *two* years. The doctor explained the severity of my journey and recovery. This made me laugh, which made him concerned since my reactions were not as they should have been. I can't begin to explain how disconnected I felt.

He went on to tell me stories of the horrible disease and its impact on past patients. He described the things that had happened to them, as he compared my recovery to theirs, I remember sinking into my seat as he spoke.

"Mohammad, you have come through a storm and you're hardly touched, but the thing with this particular disease (and the injuries your brain has sustained) is that we have no idea how it will affect you years down the line. What we do know, is that it *will* affect you."

As I left the hospital, with the worst of the storm behind me, the sunshine hit my face warmer than it ever had before.

Home sweet home

Finally, I was home, but it didn't feel like it.

I had no recollection of the decor, the layout, or the home itself. I even forgot my Mother's age, my bankcard pin number, and the *whole* year prior to my coma. To this day I cannot recall any part of 2004 before my illness.

None of that mattered, though.

I was thankful to God and my amazing family for their powerful love and guidance that brought me back to the land of the living.

I wanted to move on, but sometimes life's happenings can hold you back. This was the beginning of a new journey - a journey of a new conversation and living back on one side.

The lady with a message and the Africans in the store

Summer 2005.

My brother and I went to the city centre for a few hours. I remember getting off the number 33 bus on the corner of Corporation Street in Birmingham city centre, and as we walked up towards the Bullring, we both noticed two young ladies (identical twins) standing at the foot of the Rotunda. Feeling compelled to get closer to them, we headed over in their direction.

I felt a hand touch my shoulder, and I turned around to see an old Irish woman standing there, she said to me-

"Muhammad you were very, very ill, weren't you? But you're doing well now, aren't you? You're going to be alright, son."

She continued with "Do you have anything to hand over for the information I just gave to you?"

I reached into my pocket, pulled out a five-pound note and gave it to her. She thanked me and told

me that the twin girls were her daughters.

We made our way up to the 99p store. I was drawn to the art section and that is where I noticed a man and woman looking at me, whispering to one another. I felt paranoid and panicked, so I grabbed my brother, telling him we had to leave. As we approached the door, the man and woman stood in front of us, blocking our exit.

"Mohammad, how is everything? Are you doing well now?" the man asked in a strong West African accent. My heart skipped a beat, as I tried to make sense of a stranger seemingly knowing me.

"Don't worry about a thing. You're alright now Mohammad. You're alright," the woman said.

With that, they pivoted away. We were both shocked because of my African outburst during my time of being unwell. Maybe, there is a place between the two sides after all?

Life goes on

2019 - the year I thought I'd never see.

I feel blessed, despite still suffering many health issues as a consequence of meningitis.

I'm married to my beautiful wife Donna, and we have a daughter together - Shantaria, who is three years old. She is my ray of sunshine, my purpose.

Donna has two children - Kelsey and Tobias and they are my mountainous support. I am thankful for them every day.

Not a day goes by without me reminiscing about my experience. I'm reminded daily when my face goes into spasm, or my legs randomly collapse or how my body is still recovering/damaged. I'm reminded when my head becomes so dizzy that I have to sit down - reminded every time I make a quick turn and feel the shunt pipe pull under my skin. Although I'm left with so many issues, I am more blessed then I was before my coma.

After 16 years, I'm still trying to piece things together. Finding jigsaw pieces along the way. 2004 was the start of my jigsaw, not the end.

I'm alive, I am living, and I have found the **numbness in conversations** to put this memoir together; telling this extraordinary story from **the two sides**.

Each piece teaches me to:

Love harder,

Live the fullest life,

and embrace the sunshine after a rainy day.

RC0129826 8-

HMR 5

REGISTRATION No.	SEX	WARD
SURNAME		FIRST NAME
AGE	CONSULTANT	

REF 11101 Medtronic — LOT A44656 Medtronic Neurosurgery

REF 42823 Medtronic — LOT A47138 Medtronic Neurosurgery

OPERATION RECORD

CRANIOTOME AIR TOOL

ID No: 000451 2004/09/08 NEU2010
UHB(NHS) Trust

VENTRICULAR PERITONEAL SHUNT

ID No: 000641 2004/09/12 NEU2033
UHB(NHS) Trust

Surgeon	Anaesthetist	Theatre
HAMID / Robin Joseph	G/A Dr. ARORA	2

Operation
Insertion of delta 1.5 V.P. Shunt.

Date — Operation Notes

19/9/04 :-

- Pt positioned supine c̄ head turned to left
- Antibiotics
- Rt posterior parietal burr hole
- Peritoneum exposed in Rt hypochondrium
- Both wounds connected c̄ sub-cutaneous tunnel.
- Ventricular catheter passed into lateral ventricle 7.5 cm.
- Connected to 1.5 Delta shunt & peritoneal end placed into peritoneum.
- Valve was functioning nicely. CSF was clear under moderate pressure.
- wounds closed in layers.
- staples to skin

Post op:- Staples out after 9 days

Hamid

G 0005

RLQ1298268.

[redacted]

From: [redacted]edtronic.com>
Sent: 22 September 2016 10:56
To: [redacted]
Cc: [redacted]
Subject: Re: Medtronic Delta valve

Hi [redacted]

That product refers to our barium impregnated ventricular catheter which connects to the shunt valve and is placed in the ventricles. It is completely safe with any type of scan.

Warmest regards

[redacted]

Sent from my iPad

On 22 Sep 2016, at 10:50, [redacted]@wvt.nhs.uk> wrote:

[redacted]

In addition what is the 41101 part? Is this safe/conditional?

- Both wounds connected c̄ sub-cutaneous tunnel.
- Ventricular catheter passed into lateral ventricle 7.5 cm.
- Connected to 1.5 Delta shunt & peritoneal end placed into peritoneum.
- Valve was functioning nicely. CSF was clear with moderate pressure.
- Wounds closed in layers.
- Staples to skin

Post op:- Staples out after 9 days

[signature]

Made in the USA
Monee, IL
04 November 2026

67375614R00036